I0830190

HCG COOKBOOK

MAIN COURSE – 80 + Quick and easy to prepare at home recipes, step-by-step guide to the HCG recipes for easy weight loss

TABLE OF CONTENTS

Copyright 2018 by Noah Jerris - All rights reserved.

This document is geared towards providing exact and reliable information in regards to the topic and issue covered. The publication is sold with the idea that the publisher is not required to render accounting, officially permitted, or otherwise, qualified services. If advice is necessary, legal or professional, a practiced individual in the profession should be ordered.

- From a Declaration of Principles which was accepted and approved equally by a Committee of the American Bar Association and a Committee of Publishers and Associations.

In no way is it legal to reproduce, duplicate, or transmit any part of this document in either electronic means or in printed format. Recording of this publication is strictly prohibited and any storage of this document is not allowed unless with written permission from the publisher. All rights reserved.

The information provided herein is stated to be truthful and consistent, in that any liability, in terms of inattention or otherwise, by any usage or abuse of any policies, processes, or directions contained within is the solitary and utter responsibility of the recipient reader. Under no circumstances will any legal responsibility or blame be held against the publisher for any reparation, damages, or monetary loss due to the information herein, either directly or indirectly.

Respective authors own all copyrights not held by the publisher.

The information herein is offered for informational purposes solely, and is universal as so. The presentation of the information is without contract or any type of guarantee assurance.

The trademarks that are used are without any consent, and the publication of the trademark is without permission or backing by the trademark owner. All trademarks and brands within this book are for clarifying purposes only and are the owned by the owners themselves, not affiliated with this document.

Introduction

HCG recipes for personal enjoyment but also for family enjoyment. You will love them for sure for how easy it is to prepare them.

CHICKEN EGG ROLL

Serves:	*4*
Prep Time:	*10* Minutes
Cook Time:	*10* Minutes
Total Time:	*20* Minutes

INGREDIENTS

- 3 ½ ounces chicken breast
- 1 dash salt
- ½ packages stevia
- 3 cabbage leaves
- 1 cup shredded cabbage
- 2 Melba toast

DIRECTIONS

1. Steam the cabbage leaves for 5 minutes.
2. Add the shredded cabbage and steam for 5 minutes.
3. Place the cabbage in a bowl along with the chicken and the spices.
4. Wrap the mixture in cabbage leaves and serve topped with Melba toast.

Serves: **12**

Prep Time: **10** Minutes

Cook Time: **30** Minutes

Total Time: **40** Minutes

INGREDIENTS

- 1 cup cheese
- 8 eggs
- ¼ cup water
- 1 handful spinach
- 10 slices bacon
- ½ tbs Dijon mustard
- 1 tsp hot sauce
- Salt
- Pepper

DIRECTIONS

1. Preheat the oven to 350F.
2. Divide the spinach, cheese, and bacon into 12 greased cups of a cupcake tin.

3. Whisk together the water, eggs, mustard, hot sauce, salt, and pepper in a bowl.

4. Fill the cups with the egg mixture within 1/4 -inch from top.

5. Stir each cup, then bake for 30 minutes.

6. Serve hot.

Serves: **4**

Prep Time: **10** Minutes

Cook Time: **40** Minutes

Total Time: **50** Minutes

INGREDIENTS

- **4 eggs**
- **¾ cup cheese**
- **½ rice avocado**
- **Sour cream**
- **½ onion**
- **6 bacon strips**
- **1 can diced tomatoes**
- **½ tsp cayenne pepper**
- **4 egg whites**
- **Hot sauce**
- **½ red bell pepper**
- **½ green bell pepper**

DIRECTIONS

1. Whisk the eggs with the egg whites and cayenne
    pepper in a bowl.

2. Saute the onions, peppers and bacon until cooked.

3. Mix the tomatoes, cheese, egg and pepper mixture
    together in a baking dish.

4. Bake for 40 minutes.

5. Serve topped with avocado, sour cream and hot sauce.

Serves: **4**

Prep Time: **10**   Minutes

Cook Time: **40**   Minutes

Total Time: **50**   Minutes

INGREDIENTS

- 2 poblano chile peppers
- 12 ounces chicken sausage
- ½ tsp garlic powder
- ½ tsp onion powder
- ½ tsp salt
- 2 garlic cloves
- 12 egg whites
- 4 eggs
- 1 cup milk
- 2 tbs cilantro
- ½ tsp black pepper
- ¼ cup green onion
- 1 tsp olive oil
- ½ onion
- 4 oz. cheddar cheese

- Oil
- Sour cream
- 1 tsp hot sauce
- ½ tsp chili powder
- ½ red bell pepper

DIRECTIONS

1. Preheat the oven to 350F.
2. Roast the poblanos.
3. Place the peppers aside until cool enough to handle.
4. Peel the skin off and remove the seeds and stems.
5. Place the peppers in a greased baking dish.
6. Cook the chicken sausage until brown.
7. Remove from heat and spoon over the peppers.
8. Saute the onion and bell peppers in the oil.
9. Add the garlic and stir for a minute.
10. Spoon the mixture over the poblanos.
11. Top with the green onions and cilantro.
12. Whisk the eggs, egg whites, chili powder, onion powder, hot sauce, garlic powder, milk, salt, and pepper in a bowl.
13. Pour into baking dish, coating all of the ingredients.
14. Add cheese on top.
15. Bake for 30 minutes, remove and serve

Serves: *6*

Prep Time: *10*   Minutes

Cook Time: *40*   Minutes

Total Time: *50*   Minutes

INGREDIENTS

- 1 lb breakfast sausage
- 6 hard-boiled eggs
- ¼ cup flour
- 1 egg
- 1 ½ cups panko bread crumbs
- 4 tbs oil

DIRECTIONS

1. Preheat the oven to 350F.
2. Divide the sausage into 6 portions.
3. Wrap the eggs with the sausage.
4. Roll them into flour, egg wash, and panko crumbs in this order.
5. Preheat the oil in a pan.
6. Cook the balls until brown on all sides.

7. Place on a tray.

8. Bake for 25 minutes, remove and serve

Serves: **4**

Prep Time: **10**   Minutes

Cook Time: **10**   Minutes

Total Time: **20**   Minutes

INGREDIENTS

- 1 egg
- 6 tbs egg whites
- ¼ spinach
- 3 tbs green onion
- Salt
- Pepper

DIRECTIONS

1. Preheat the burner.
2. Grease a skillet with cooking spray.
3. Crack the egg into the skillet and add 6 tbs egg whites.

Serves: *8*

Prep Time: *10* Minutes

Cook Time: *15* Minutes

Total Time: *25* Minutes

INGREDIENTS

- 1 egg
- ½ tsp vanilla
- ½ tsp baking powder
- Salt
- ½ tsp flour
- Cinnamon
- Stevia
- ½ cup water

DIRECTIONS

1. Mix all of the ingredients and form a batter.
2. Fry in coconut oil.
3. Serve with your favorite toppings.

Serves: *12*

Prep Time: *10*   Minutes

Cook Time: *30*   Minutes

Total Time: *40*   Minutes

INGREDIENTS

- Vegetables
- Meat
- 1 ½ tsp seasoning
- 12 eggs
- 12 muffin tin liners
- 1 cup cheese

DIRECTIONS

1. Place the diced meat and vegetables and cheese in the bottom of the muffin cups.
2. Beat the eggs and season in a bowl.
3. Pour the eggs into the cups and bake for 30 minutes.
4. Serve hot.

Serves: *1*

Prep Time: *5*   Minutes

Cook Time: *5*   Minutes

Total Time: *10*   Minutes

INGREDIENTS

- 2 toast
- ½ tsp cilantro
- Pepper
- 1 egg white
- 1 tsp salsa
- 2 tbs water
- Salt

DIRECTIONS

1. Cook the egg white in a pan, then season with salt and pepper and add 1 tbs water.
2. Cook for ½ minute covered.
3. Divide in 2 and place each half on the toast.
4. Top with salsa and cilantro.

Serves: *1*

Prep Time: *5*   Minutes

Cook Time: *5*   Minutes

Total Time: *10*   Minutes

INGREDIENTS

- 5 tbs salsa
- 1 egg
- 5 tbs egg substitute
- Salt
- Pepper

DIRECTIONS

1. Scramble the eggs.
2. Add the egg substitute and cook.
3. Season with salt and pepper.
4. Serve topped with salsa.

Serves: *2*
Prep Time: *5*   Minutes

Cook Time: *10*   Minutes

Total Time: *15*   Minutes

INGREDIENTS

- 1 egg
- 2 egg whites
- Cheese
- Salt
- Red pepper
- Tomatoes
- Milk
- Mushrooms
- Pepper
- Green pepper

DIRECTIONS

1. Whisk the eggs, egg whites, and milk together.
2. Cook in a skillet for 3 minutes.

3.   When almost set, top with the vegetables and add
     cheese on top.

4.   Serve immediately.

Serves: *4*

Prep Time: *10*   Minutes

Cook Time: *10*   Minutes

Total Time: *20*   Minutes

INGREDIENTS

- 1 egg
- 2 cups berries
- 2 tsp baking soda
- 2 cups Greek yogurt
- ½ tsp salt
- 1 tsp vanilla
- 2 ½ tbs maple syrup
- 1 ½ cup flour

DIRECTIONS

1. Mix well the ingredients in a bowl.
2. Cook the pancakes in a skillet for 3 minutes on each side.
3. Serve topped with maple syrup.

Serves: **6**
Prep Time: **5**   Minutes

Cook Time: **15**   Minutes

Total Time: **20**   Minutes

INGREDIENTS

- 6 tbs milk
- 3 tbs water
- 3 tbs mayonnaise
- 1 cup flour

DIRECTIONS

1. Mix the ingredients except for the mayo in a bowl.
2. Add in the mayonnaise and mix.
3. Stir in the water and milk.
4. Form balls and place on a baking sheet.
5. Bake for 15 minutes.
6. Serve immediately.

Serves: *4*

Prep Time: *10* Minutes

Cook Time: *10* Minutes

Total Time: *20* Minutes

INGREDIENTS

- Bread slices
- Egg substitute
- 1 tsp cinnamon
- Stevia
- 1 tsp vanilla
- Butter

DIRECTIONS

1. Mix the egg substitute, vanilla, and cinnamon in a bowl.
2. Melt the butter in a skillet.
3. Coat the bread slices with the egg mixture.
4. Cook until golden.
5. Serve immediately.

Serves: *2*
Prep Time: *10*   Minutes

Cook Time: *10*   Minutes

Total Time: *20*   Minutes

INGREDIENTS

- 6 eggs
- 1 ½ cups bell peppers
- 1 onion
- Salt
- Pepper
- Thyme
- 1 can potatoes

DIRECTIONS

1. Whisk the eggs together in a bowl.
2. Season and add the vegetables.
3. Cook until fluffy.
4. Serve hot.

Serves: *4*
Prep Time: *10*   Minutes

Cook Time: *30*   Minutes

Total Time: *40*   Minutes

INGREDIENTS

Cake
- 1 egg
- 1 cup flour
- 1 tsp baking soda
- ½ cup yogurt
- ½ cup apple sauce
- 1 cup brown sugar
- 1 tsp vanilla
- 1 ½ cups apple cored

Topping
- 3 tbs brown sugar
- 3 tbs flour
- 1 tbs butter

DIRECTIONS

1. Mix all of the cake ingredients in a bowl.
2. Place on a baking sheet.

3.   Mix the topping ingredients, then add over the cake.

4.   Bake for 30 minutes.

5.   Allow to cool, then serve.

Serves: *12*

Prep Time: *5* Minutes

Cook Time: *25* Minutes

Total Time: *30* Minutes

INGREDIENTS

- 1 ½ cups flour
- 1 tsp baking soda
- 1/8 tsp cloves
- 1 cup brown sugar
- 1 cup pumpkin puree
- 1 tsp ginger
- 1/3 cup milk
- 1 egg
- 2 tbs oil
- ½ cup cranberries
- ½ tsp cinnamon
- 1/3 tsp baking powder
- Salt

DIRECTIONS

1. Pulse all of the ingredients in a food processor.

2. Pour the batter into 12 muffin cups.

3. Bake for 25 minutes.

4. Serve warm.

Serves: **2**
Prep Time: **10**   Minutes

Cook Time: **20**   Minutes

Total Time: **30**   Minutes

INGREDIENTS

- 2 tbs water
- 1 tbs brown sugar
- ¼ cup coconut flakes
- 1 cup bananas
- ½ cup quinoa
- ¾ cup coconut milk
- 1 cup strawberries

DIRECTIONS

1. Cook the quinoa.
2. When half done, add the coconut milk and sugar and mix well.
3. Cook until done.
4. Toast the coconut flakes.
5. Serve topped with fruits and flakes.

Serves: *2*

Prep Time: *10*   Minutes

Cook Time: *10*   Minutes

Total Time: *20*   Minutes

INGREDIENTS

- 2 tortillas
- 2 cups spinach leaves
- 4 eggs
- Oil
- 1 tsp cumin
- Cilantro
- Hot sauce
- 1 tsp turmeric
- ½ cup beans
- Salt
- Pepper

DIRECTIONS

1. Cook the beans with the hot sauce and spices.
2. Garnish with cilantro.

3. Fry the spinach leaves.

4. Scramble the eggs.

5. Add the beans, eggs and spinach leaves on the tortillas.

6. Serve topped with avocado slices and garnished with cilantro.

Serves: *2*
Prep Time: *5*   Minutes

Cook Time: *10*   Minutes

Total Time: *15*   Minutes

INGREDIENTS

- 2 cups blueberries
- 1 tsp lemon rind
- 1 tbs lemon juice
- 1 cup oats
- ¼ cup brown sugar
- ½ tsp cinnamon powder
- 4 cups water
- Salt

DIRECTIONS

1. Prepare the compote.
2. Prepare the oats.
3. Serve the oats with the compote.

SPICY SHRIMP STIR FRY

Serves: *1*

Prep Time: *10*   Minutes

Cook Time: *10*   Minutes

Total Time: *20*   Minutes

INGREDIENTS

- 1 orange
- Cayenne powder
- 3 oz shrimp
- Ginger powder
- 4 tbs vegetable stock
- Curry powder
- 25 cups red onion
- 1 cup cabbage
- Garlic powder

DIRECTIONS

1. **Coat the shrimp in the seasonings.**

2. Pour the broth into a pan, then add cabbage, onion, and shrimp.

3. Cook until the shrimp turns pink.

4. Serve topped with orange juice and orange slices.

Serves: **4**

Prep Time: **10**   Minutes

Cook Time: **30**   Minutes

Total Time: **40**   Minutes

INGREDIENTS

- 1 garlic clove
- 2 tsp chili powder
- 4 cups chicken broth
- 2 tsp cayenne
- 4 tsp cumin
- 1 cup tomatoes
- 2 tsp onion powder
- 1 lb chicken
- ¼ cup cilantro

DIRECTIONS

1. Preheat a pot.
2. Cook the garlic for 5 minutes.
3. Add tomatoes, chicken broth, onion powder, cumin, chili powder, and cayenne.

4. Bring to a boil, then reduce to a simmer.

5. Add the chicken, simmer for 20 minutes and stir in the cilantro and simmer for another 5 minutes.

6. Serve immediately.

Serves: *4*

Prep Time: *10*   Minutes

Cook Time: *30*   Minutes

Total Time: *40*   Minutes

INGREDIENTS

- 2 cloves garlic
- ½ lb Beef Sirloin steaks
- Chicken broth
- 2 tbs liquid Aminos
- 1 tsp onion powder
- 1 tbs parsley
- 2 cups broccoli florets

DIRECTIONS

1. Sauté the beef in a few tbs of chicken broth until brown.
2. Add onion powder, garlic, broccoli, liquid aminos and parsley.
3. Saute until well done.
4. Serve immediately.

Serves: *1*

Prep Time: *5*   Minutes

Cook Time: *15*   Minutes

Total Time: *20*   Minutes

INGREDIENTS

- 2 cloves garlic
- Salt
- Pepper
- 3 stalks celery
- 3 oz chicken tenders
- 4 cups chicken broth
- 4 slices ginger

DIRECTIONS

1. Bring the broth to a boil.
2. Add the garlic, ginger, and celery.
3. Simmer for 5 minutes.
4. Add in the chicken and boil for 10 more minutes.
5. Season with salt and pepper.
6. Serve immediately.

Serves: **4**

Prep Time: **10**   Minutes

Cook Time: **10**   Minutes

Total Time: **20**   Minutes

INGREDIENTS

- 1 lb chicken breast
- 8 cups cabbage
- 1 onion
- 8 cups chicken broth
- 1 zucchini
- 2 egg whites
- ¼ soy sauce
- 1 clove garlic
- ¼ tsp white pepper
- Salt

DIRECTIONS

1. Pour the broth, pepper, salt and soy sauce in a pot, then bring to a boil.

2. Drizzle the lightly beaten egg whites slowly into the broth, stirring constantly.

3. Add the zucchini, garlic, onion and cabbage.

4. Reduce to a simmer, until cabbage is tender, then add cooked chicken.

5. Cook for another 2 minutes.

6. Serve immediately.

Serves: **1**

Prep Time: **10** Minutes

Cook Time: **10** Minutes

Total Time: **20** Minutes

INGREDIENTS

- 1 tsp dill
- 2 tbs white onion
- 2 tbs lemon juice
- 1 cup chicken broth
- 5 stems asparagus
- ½ tsp onion powder
- Salt
- Pepper

DIRECTIONS

1. Steam the asparagus until tender.
2. Pulse the asparagus, onion and puree in a blender until smooth.
3. Cook the mixture along with the other ingredients until warmed throughout, and serve.

Serves: **4**

Prep Time: **10** Minutes

Cook Time: **50** Minutes

Total Time: **60** Minutes

INGREDIENTS

- 2 cloves garlic
- 1 ¼ cup celery
- 100g steak
- 1 ½ cups beef broth
- 2 tbs onion
- ½ tsp garlic powder
- ½ tsp rosemary
- 1 bay leaf
- Salt
- Pepper

DIRECTIONS

1. Slice the meat and season with salt, pepper, and garlic powder.
2. Saute the steak, diced onion and garlic until brown.

3.   Add the rest of the ingredients and simmer for 45
     minutes.

4.   Season and serve.

Serves: *1*

Prep Time: *10*   Minutes

Cook Time: *15*   Minutes

Total Time: *25*   Minutes

INGREDIENTS

- 1 ½ cups vegetable
- 2 tbs onion
- 100 g crab
- 1 ½ tomatoes
- 1 garlic clove
- 2 tsp seasoning
- Salt
- Pepper

DIRECTIONS

1. Place all of the ingredients in a pot.
2. Bring to a boil, then reduce heat and simmer for 15 minutes.
3. Serve hot.

Serves: **1**

Prep Time: **10** Minutes

Cook Time: **20** Minutes

Total Time: **30** Minutes

INGREDIENTS

- **100g**
- **1 clove garlic**
- **2 cups chicken broth**
- **2 tbs lemon juice**
- **2 tbs onion**
- **3 tsp curry**
- **Salt**
- **Pepper**

DIRECTIONS

1. **Sauté the chicken, onion, lemon juice and garlic in a pan until well done.**
2. **Remove the chicken and shred it.**
3. **Place the rest of the ingredients in the pan, along with the chicken.**

Serves: *1*
Prep Time: *5*   Minutes

Cook Time: *10*   Minutes

Total Time: *15*   Minutes

INGREDIENTS

- ¾ cup chicken broth
- 2 tbs tomato paste
- 2 tbs milk
- ½ cup tomatoes
- 1 tbs vinegar
- 1 tbs onion
- 1 clove garlic
- 1 tsp oregano
- Salt
- Pepper
- Basil leaves

DIRECTIONS

1. **Pulse the ingredients in a food processor, saving the basil for garnish.**

2. Cook the mixture until heated.
3. Serve garnished with basil leaves and toast.

Serves: *1*

Prep Time: *5*   Minutes

Cook Time: *10*   Minutes

Total Time: *15*   Minutes

INGREDIENTS

- ½ cup celery
- 1 tbs vinegar
- 1 tsp seasoning
- 100 g crab
- Red pepper flakes
- 2 tbs lemon juice
- 2 tbs onion

DIRECTIONS

1. Sauté the ingredients in a pan until celery is tender.
2. Season to taste.
3. Serve over toast.

Serves: *1*

Prep Time: 5   Minutes

Cook Time: 5   Minutes

Total Time: *10*   Minutes

INGREDIENTS

- ½ cup orange segments
- 1 packet stevia
- 1 toast
- 100g chicken breast
- ¼ tsp salt
- Orange citrus dressing
- 2 cups romaine lettuce

DIRECTIONS

1. Cook the chicken in a skillet until golden.
2. Combine all of the ingredients in a bowl.
3. Serve immediately.

Serves: **1**

Prep Time: **5** Minutes

Cook Time: **10** Minutes

Total Time: **15** Minutes

INGREDIENTS

- 100g chicken
- ½ tsp onion powder
- ½ tsp garlic powder
- ½ tsp oregano
- 1 tsp paprika
- ½ tsp thyme
- ½ tsp black pepper
- ¼ tsp salad greens

DIRECTIONS

1. Rub the chicken with the combined spices.
2. Grill the pink until golden.
3. Serve over the salad greens and desired dressing.

Serves: *1*

Prep Time: *5* Minutes

Cook Time: *0* Minutes

Total Time: *5* Minutes

INGREDIENTS

- ¼ tsp salt
- 2 tsp parsley
- ¼ cup vinegar
- 2 tsp green onion
- Pepper
- Stevia
- 1 cucumber

DIRECTIONS

1. Chop the cucumber.
2. Mix the ingredients in a bowl.
3. Refrigerate for at least 10 minutes, then serve.

Serves: *1*
Prep Time: *10*   Minutes

Cook Time: *0*   Minutes

Total Time: *10*   Minutes

INGREDIENTS

- 2 tbs apple vinegar
- Grapefruit juice
- ½ tsp ginger
- Salt
- 1 red grapefruit
- 1 cucumber
- Pepper
- Cilantro
- 2 tbs onion
- Ruby red dressing

DIRECTIONS

1. Peel the grapefruit and cut it into cubes.
2. Mix with the rest of the ingredients and season.
3. Serve topped with red dressing.

Serves: **2**

Prep Time: **5**   Minutes

Cook Time: **0**   Minutes

Total Time: **5**   Minutes

INGREDIENTS

- ½ cup green apple
- 1 tbs lemon juice
- Salt
- Pepper
- Stevia
- ½ cup cucumber
- 2 tbs apple cider vinegar

DIRECTIONS

1. Chop the apple and cucumber.
2. Combine the ingredients and add stevia.
3. Serve immediately.

Serves: **1**

Prep Time: **10** Minutes

Cook Time: **0** Minutes

Total Time: **10** Minutes

INGREDIENTS

- 1 ½ cups cabbage
- ¼ tsp onion powder
- Cayenne pepper
- Salt
- Pepper
- 2 tbs vinegar
- 2 tbs lemon juice
- 1 tsp horseradish
- 1 clove garlic
- ½ tsp mustard

DIRECTIONS

1. Slice the cabbage.
2. Mix the rest of the ingredients in a bowl.
3. Pour the mixture over the cabbage and serve.

Serves: *1*
Prep Time: *5* Minutes

Cook Time: *5* Minutes

Total Time: *10* Minutes

INGREDIENTS

- 100g lobster
- 1 serving Tarragon Vinaigrette
- 2 tbs lemon juice
- 1 tbs tarragon
- ½ tsp garlic powder
- 2 tbs onion
- 1 tbs green onion

DIRECTIONS

1. Cook the lobster.
2. Sauté the lobster, lemon juice, green onion, onion, tarragon, garlic powder, salt, and pepper until onion is tender.
3. Top the lettuce with the lobster mixture.
4. Serve topped with Tarragon Vinaigrette.

Serves: **1**

Prep Time: **10** Minutes

Cook Time: **20** Minutes

Total Time: **30** Minutes

INGREDIENTS

- 2 tbs lemon juice
- 1 tbs onion
- 1 tbs parsley
- Salt
- Radishes
- Pepper

DIRECTIONS

1. Combine all of the ingredients in a bowl.
2. Refrigerate for at least 20 minutes.
3. Serve.

Serves: *1*

Prep Time: *5*   Minutes

Cook Time: *5*   Minutes

Total Time: *10*   Minutes

INGREDIENTS

- 1 bunch spinach
- Pepper
- Mint leaves
- 2 tbs vinegar
- 2 tbs lemon juice
- 5 strawberries
- ¼ tsp Stevia
- Salt

DIRECTIONS

1. Blend 2 strawberries, lemon juice, vinegar, Stevia, salt, and pepper together.
2. Pour the dressing over the salad and the sliced remained strawberry.
3. Serve topped with mint leaves.

CILANTRO SKEWERS

Serves: *1*

Prep Time: *20*   Minutes

Cook Time: *120*   Minutes

Total Time: *140*   Minutes

INGREDIENTS

- Cherry tomatoes
- Red pepper flakes
- Salt
- Pepper
- 2 tbs lemon juice
- Cilantro
- 100g shrimp

DIRECTIONS

1. Mix the cilantro, red pepper flakes, salt, pepper and shrimp together.
2. Marinade for at least 2 hours.
3. Place on skewers alternating with tomatoes.

4. Cook on a barbeque.
5. Season with salt and pepper.
6. Serve immediately.

Serves: *14*
Prep Time: *10*   Minutes

Cook Time: *10*   Minutes

Total Time: *20*   Minutes

INGREDIENTS

- 1/8 cup water
- 100g shrimp
- 1 onion
- Pepper
- 1/ tsp curry powder
- ¼ tsp cumin
- Salt
- 4 garlic cloves

DIRECTIONS

1. Cook the garlic and onion until translucent.
2. Add in the shrimp, seasonings and water.
3. Cook until done.
4. Serve immediately.

Serves: *1*

Prep Time: *10*   Minutes

Cook Time: *15*   Minutes

Total Time: *25*   Minutes

INGREDIENTS

- 100g orange roughy fillet
- 2 tbs lemon juice
- 1 tsp thyme
- 1 tsp rosemary
- ¼ tsp onion powder
- Salt
- Pepper

DIRECTIONS

1. **Place the ingredients in a baking dish and cover with tin foil.**
2. **Bake at 350F for 15 minutes.**
3. **Serve hot.**

Serves: **1**

Prep Time: **10** Minutes

Cook Time: **20** Minutes

Total Time: **30** Minutes

INGREDIENTS

- ¼ cup lemon juice
- 1 lemon zest
- 100g tilapia
- 1 tbs onion
- 1 tsp dill
- Salt
- Pepper

DIRECTIONS

1. Place the ingredients in a tin foil, then wrap them up.
2. Cook on a grill until done
3. Serve when ready

Serves: *1*
Prep Time: *10*   Minutes

Cook Time: *10*   Minutes

Total Time: *20*   Minutes

INGREDIENTS

- 100g sea Bass
- 2 cloves garlic
- 1 lemon juice
- 1 lemon zest
- 1 tbs onion
- ½ tsp parsley
- Salt
- Pepper

DIRECTIONS

1. Place the ingredients in a tin foil bag.
2. Cook on the barbeque for 10 minutes.
3. Serve topped with fresh parsley.

Serves: *1*
Prep Time: *10*   Minutes

Cook Time: *5*   Minutes

Total Time: *15*   Minutes

INGREDIENTS

- ½ tsp ginger
- 100g whitefish
- 1 tbs mustard
- 1 tsp wasabi powder

DIRECTIONS

1. Mix the mustard with the wasabi powder.
2. Add the ginger.
3. Coat the fish with the mixture.
4. Allow to sit for at least half an hour.
5. Grill for 5 minutes.
6. Serve hot.

Serves: *1*

Prep Time: *5*   Minutes

Cook Time: *25*   Minutes

Total Time: *30*   Minutes

INGREDIENTS

- ½ tbs milk
- ½ tsp Cajun seasoning
- 100g chicken

DIRECTIONS

1. Preheat the oven to 350F.
2. Coat the chicken with milk.
3. Sprinkle with Cajun seasoning.
4. Bake for 25 minutes.
5. Serve immediately.

Serves: *1*

Prep Time: *5*   Minutes

Cook Time: *0*   Minutes

Total Time: *5*   Minutes

INGREDIENTS

- ½ tomato
- 1 toast
- 100g chicken
- Basil
- Salt
- Pepper

DIRECTIONS

1. Cook the chicken, allow to chill, then shred.
2. Arrange the ingredients on top of the toast.
3. Serve immediately.

Serves: *1*

Prep Time: *10*   Minutes

Cook Time: *25*   Minutes

Total Time: *35*   Minutes

INGREDIENTS

- ½ tsp oregano
- Parsley
- 100g chicken
- 1 toast
- ½ tsp basil
- 3 garlic cloves
- 2 tsp onion
- Salt
- Pepper

DIRECTIONS

1. Crush the toast and combine with oregano, basil, salt, and pepper.
2. Coat the chicken with the mixture and place in a casserole dish.

3. Cook covered for 25 minutes at 375F.

4. Serve topped with marinara sauce and parsley.

Serves: *1*
Prep Time: *10*   Minutes

Cook Time: *30*   Minutes

Total Time: *40*   Minutes

INGREDIENTS

- 100g chicken
- 2 garlic cloves
- ½ tsp salt
- ½ onion
- 1 cup chicken broth
- Black pepper
- Curry powder

DIRECTIONS

1. Sauté the onion and garlic in the lemon juice.
2. Stir in the curry powder and salt and mix well.
3. Add the chicken and the broth in the pan.
4. Cook for 30 minutes.
5. Serve topped with black pepper.

Serves: *1*

Prep Time: *10*   Minutes

Cook Time: *30*   Minutes

Total Time: *40*   Minutes

INGREDIENTS

- 100g chicken
- BBQ sauce
- 1 tsp oregano
- 1 tsp onion powder 1 toast
- 1 tsp garlic powder
- Salt
- Pepper

DIRECTIONS

1. Crush the toast and mix with onion powder, garlic powder, oregano, salt and pepper.
2. Coat the chicken in the mixture.
3. Bake covered with tin foil and 350F for 30 minutes.
4. Cook 5 more minutes uncovered.
5. Serve topped with BBQ sauce.

Serves: *1*

Prep Time: *10*   Minutes

Cook Time: *30*   Minutes

Total Time: *40*   Minutes

INGREDIENTS

- ½ lemon juice
- Black pepper
- 3 tbs onion
- 100g chicken
- 5 garlic cloves

DIRECTIONS

1. Preheat the oven to 350F.
2. Cook the onion in a saucepan until tender.
3. Transfer to a baking dish and place the chicken on top.
4. Pour lemon juice and black pepper over.
5. Add the garlic cloves over and cover with aluminum foil.
6. Cook for 30 minutes, then serve.

Serves: **1**

Prep Time: **10** Minutes

Cook Time: **10** Minutes

Total Time: **20** Minutes

INGREDIENTS

- 100g chicken
- 2 tbs lemon juice
- ¼ tsp nutmeg
- ¼ tsp cinnamon
- Salt
- Pepper
- 1/8 tsp cloves
- 1/8 tsp allspice

DIRECTIONS

1. Mix the cloves, cinnamon, allspice, nutmeg, salt, and pepper in a bowl.
2. Rub the chicken with the mixture and place in a skillet with the lemon juice.
3. Grill until well done, and serve.

Serves: **1**

Prep Time: **10**   Minutes

Cook Time: **15**   Minutes

Total Time: **25**   Minutes

INGREDIENTS

- **2 garlic cloves**
- **2 tbs lemon juice**
- **2 tbs onion**
- **100g lean hamburger**
- **2 tbs basil**
- **Worcestershire sauce**
- **Garlic powder**
- **Salt**
- **Pepper**
- **½ apple**
- **2 tbs green onion**

DIRECTIONS

1. **Sauté the chopped apple, green onion, onion, and garlic in the lemon juice.**

2. Add the basil when almost done.

3. Mix the hamburger, Worcestershire, apple mixture, garlic and onion powders, salt and pepper.

4. Grill the burger until well done.

Serves: *1*
Prep Time: *10*   Minutes

Cook Time: *15*   Minutes

Total Time: *20*   Minutes

INGREDIENTS

- 100g lean steak
- Onion powder
- Salt
- Pepper
- 1 onion
- Garlic powder

DIRECTIONS

1. Cut the steak and season with garlic and onion powders.
2. Slide the beef and onion wedges onto skewers.
3. Season with salt and pepper.
4. Cook on a barbeque.
5. Serve immediately.

Serves: **1**

Prep Time: **10** Minutes

Cook Time: **20** Minutes

Total Time: **30** Minutes

INGREDIENTS

- **1 sprig rosemary**
- **Salt**
- **2 tbs lemon juice**
- **100g veal**
- **2 cloves garlic**
- **Pepper**
- **2 tbs apple cider vinegar**
- **½ tsp onion powder**

DIRECTIONS

1. **Combine the ingredients in a zip lock bag.**
2. **Marinate for 4 hours.**
3. **Cook in a pan until well done.**
4. **Serve topped with the remaining sauce.**

Serves: *1*
Prep Time: *10* Minutes

Cook Time: *20* Minutes

Total Time: *30* Minutes

INGREDIENTS

- ½ tsp red pepper
- 100g steak
- 1 tbs rice vinegar
- 1 tbs rosemary
- 5 minced cloves garlic

DIRECTIONS

1. Coat the steak in the rice vinegar.
2. Rub the steak with the mixed seasonings.
3. Refrigerate covered for at least 4 hours.
4. Cook on the grill.
5. Serve hot.

Serves: *1*

Prep Time: *10*   Minutes

Cook Time: *15*   Minutes

Total Time: *25*   Minutes

INGREDIENTS

- Worcestershire sauce
- Basil
- 2 garlic cloves
- 100g chicken breast
- 2 tbs onion
- Salt
- Pepper

DIRECTIONS

1. Mix all of the ingredients.
2. Cook the patty on both sides until well done.

Serves: *4*

Prep Time: *10*   Minutes

Cook Time: *20*   Minutes

Total Time: *30*   Minutes

INGREDIENTS

Steak

- **100g lean steak**
- **Garlic powder**
- **Pepper**
- **2 tbs lemon juice**
- **Salt**

Sauce

- **1 clove garlic**
- **½ tsp mustard**
- **½ tsp onion powder**
- **¼ cup ketchup**
- **Cayenne pepper**
- **Salt**
- **2 tbs apple cider vinegar**
- **2 tsp onion**

DIRECTIONS

1. Cut the steak into cubes, season with garlic
    powder, salt and pepper and saute in a pan.

2. Mix the sauce ingredients in a bowl.

3. Serve the steak covered in the sauce.

Serves: *1*

Prep Time: *10*   Minutes

Cook Time: *10*   Minutes

Total Time: *20*   Minutes

INGREDIENTS

- 100g lean ground veal
- ¼ cup tomato paste
- 1 garlic clove
- Worcestershire sauce
- 1 toast
- 2 tbs onion
- ½ tsp parsley
- 1 tsp oregano
- ½ tsp salt
- ½ tsp black pepper

DIRECTIONS

1. Mix the ingredients together in a bowl.
2. Form balls from the mixture.
3. Cook in a covered dish at 350F for 15 minutes.

BAKED APPLES

Serves: *1*

Prep Time: *10*   Minutes

Cook Time: *30*   Minutes

Total Time: *40*   Minutes

INGREDIENTS

- 1/8 tsp cloves
- Salt
- 1 lemon juice
- 1 lemon zest
- 1 apple
- ½ tsp cinnamon
- ¼ tsp nutmeg

DIRECTIONS

1. Place cored apple in a dish and squeeze lemon juice inside and around it.
2. Mix the remaining ingredients and repeat.
3. Top with lemon zest.
4. Bake at 350F for 30 minutes, allow to chill and serve

Serves: *1*

Prep Time: *5*   Minutes

Cook Time: *10*   Minutes

Total Time: *15*   Minutes

INGREDIENTS

- 1 apple
- 1/8 tsp cloves
- Salt
- Stevia
- 1 tsp cinnamon
- 1 lemon juice
- ¼ tsp nutmeg

DIRECTIONS

1. Coat the apples with the ingredients.
2. Place in a pan along with the lemon juice and grill until tender.
3. Serve warm.

Serves: *1*

Prep Time: *5*   Minutes

Cook Time: *0*   Minutes

Total Time: *5*   Minutes

INGREDIENTS

- 3 ½ oz cottage cheese
- 1 orange zest
- Stevia
- 1 orange

DIRECTIONS

1. Mix the ingredients together in a bowl.
2. Serve immediately.

Serves: *1*

Prep Time: *5*   Minutes

Cook Time: *0*   Minutes

Total Time: *5*   Minutes

INGREDIENTS

- **Strawberries**
- **4 drops vanilla crème Stevia**
- **1 packet powdered Stevia**
- **1 tbs milk**

DIRECTIONS

1. **Toss the sliced strawberries with the rest of the ingredients.**
2. **Serve immediately.**

Serves: *1*

Prep Time: *5*   Minutes

Cook Time: *5*   Minutes

Total Time: *10*   Minutes

INGREDIENTS

- Powdered Stevia
- Cinnamon
- 1 grapefruit

DIRECTIONS

1. Peel the grapefruit and cut into cubes.
2. Toss in the Stevia and cinnamon.
3. Cook under the broiler for 5 minutes.
4. Serve warm.

Serves: *1*

Prep Time: *5*   Minutes

Cook Time: *0*   Minutes

Total Time: *5*   Minutes

INGREDIENTS

- Ice cubes
- 2 strawberries
- ½ lemon juice
- 8 oz sparkling mineral water
- Lemon zest
- Stevia

DIRECTIONS

1. Mix the ingredients and stir to combine until the strawberries are mashed.
2. Serve over ice cubes.

Serves: *1*
Prep Time: *5*   Minutes

Cook Time: *0*   Minutes

Total Time: *5*   Minutes

INGREDIENTS

- Stevia
- Ice cubes
- ½ grapefruit juice
- 8 oz sparkling mineral water

DIRECTIONS

1. Mix the grapefruit juice with the water.
2. Pour over the ice cubes and serve.

Serves: *1*

Prep Time: *5* Minutes

Cook Time: *0* Minutes

Total Time: *5* Minutes

INGREDIENTS

- Vanilla stevia
- Ice cubes
- 1 peeled orange
- 1 orange zest
- 2 tbs milk

DIRECTIONS

1. Blend all of the ingredients together.
2. Serve immediately.

Serves: *1*

Prep Time: *5*   Minutes

Cook Time: *0*   Minutes

Total Time: *5*   Minutes

INGREDIENTS

- Lemon stevia
- Ice cubes
- 5 strawberries
- ¼ lemon
- 2 tbs milk

DIRECTIONS

1. Blend the ingredients until smooth.
2. Serve immediately.

Serves: *1*
Prep Time: *5*   Minutes

Cook Time: *0*   Minutes

Total Time: *5*   Minutes

INGREDIENTS

- **Chocolate stevia**
- **Ice cubes**
- **5 strawberries**
- **2 tbs milk**
- **½ tsp cocoa powder**

DIRECTIONS

1. **Blend the ingredients until smooth.**
2. **Serve immediately.**

Serves: **4**

Prep Time: **5**   Minutes

Cook Time: **0**   Minutes

Total Time: **5**   Minutes

INGREDIENTS

- 1 cup almonds
- ¼ cup walnuts
- ¼ cup cashews
- 1 tbs ground coffee beans
- 1 ¼ cup medjool dates
- 2 tbs cocoa powder
- ¼ tsp vanilla extract

DIRECTIONS

1. Pulse the ingredients in a food processor.
2. Spread into a baking dish and refrigerate for at least 1 hour.
3. Cut into bars and serve.

Serves: *12*
Prep Time: *5*   Minutes

Cook Time: *0*   Minutes

Total Time: *5*   Minutes

INGREDIENTS

- 1 tsp vanilla
- 3 tbs chocolate chips
- 2 cups raw cashews
- 2 cups medjool dates

DIRECTIONS

1. Pulse the cashews, then add dates.
2. Add vanilla and pulse again.
3. Fold in the chocolate chips.
4. Form the cookies and refrigerate for at least 30 minutes.
5. Serve.

Serves: *12*

Prep Time: *5*   Minutes

Cook Time: *0*   Minutes

Total Time: *5*   Minutes

INGREDIENTS

- ½ cup dried bananas
- 1/8 cup water
- 1 cup dates
- 2 cups peanuts

DIRECTIONS

1. Pulse the ingredients in a food processor until a dough forms.
2. Form the cookies in desired shapes.
3. Store in the fridge.

Serves: **4**
Prep Time: **5**   Minutes

Cook Time: **45**   Minutes

Total Time: **50**   Minutes

INGREDIENTS

- ½ tsp pepper
- 1 head cauliflower
- 2 tbs oil
- 1 ½ tsp paprika
- ½ tsp chili powder
- ½ tsp mesquite seasoning
- 1 tsp salt

DIRECTIONS

1. Preheat the oven to 425F.
2. Mix the spices together.
3. Coat the cauliflower with oil and seasonings.
4. Bake on a baking sheet for 30 minutes.
5. Serve cold.

Serves: **4**

Prep Time: **5** Minutes

Cook Time: **5** Minutes

Total Time: **10** Minutes

INGREDIENTS

- 4 oz apple sauce
- 2 tsp sugar
- 2 cups rhubarb

DIRECTIONS

1. Cut the rhubarb in small pieces.
2. Soften the rhubarb in the microwave.
3. Mix the apple sauce and sugar.
4. Pour the mixture and the rhubarb into popsicle molds.
5. Freeze overnight, then serve.

Serves: **4**

Prep Time: **5**   Minutes

Cook Time: **10**   Minutes

Total Time: **15**   Minutes

INGREDIENTS

- 1 zucchini
- Salt
- Pepper

DIRECTIONS

1. **Cut the zucchini into slices, then pat them dry.**
2. **Bake them on a lined baking sheet in the preheated oven at 450F for 10 minutes.**
3. **Flip over and bake for another 10 minutes.**

Serves: **4**

Prep Time: **5**   Minutes

Cook Time: **2**   Minutes

Total Time: **7**   Minutes

INGREDIENTS

- 1 cup water
- 1 cup yogurt
- 1 package Jello

DIRECTIONS

1. Dissolve the Jello in the boiling water.
2. Stir the Jello mixture in the yogurt.
3. Refrigerate until set, then serve.

Serves: **4**

Prep Time: **15** Minutes

Cook Time: **0** Minutes

Total Time: **15** Minutes

INGREDIENTS

- 1 cup whip light
- 1 box instant chocolate pudding
- 1 cups milk
- 1 packages oreo
- 4 blocks chocolate bar

DIRECTIONS

1. Mix the pudding mix with the milk.
2. Crush the oreos.
3. Place one package into the pudding.
4. Chop 2 blocks of chocolate and stir in the pudding.
5. Serve topped with the other crushed oreo package

Serves: *14*

Prep Time: *10*   Minutes

Cook Time: *0*   Minutes

Total Time: *10*   Minutes

INGREDIENTS

- 2 cups graham snacks
- 1 cup fruit mix
- 4 cups popcorn

DIRECTIONS

1. Mix all of the ingredients together in a bowl.
2. Serve.

Serves: *16*

Prep Time: *5*   Minutes

Cook Time: *0*   Minutes

Total Time: *5*   Minutes

INGREDIENTS

- ½ cup almond butter
- ½ cup water
- 1 cup chocolate powder
- 6 packets stevia
- 2 tbs almond meal
- ½ cup cocoa powder
- ¼ cup flax seeds

DIRECTIONS

1. Mix the almond butter with the water.
2. Add the remaining ingredients except for the almond meal.
3. Mix until a dough is formed.
4. Cut into 16 pieces.
5. Serve.

www.ingramcontent.com/pod-product-compliance
Lightning Source LLC
Chambersburg PA
CBHW031255250726
48655CB00005B/2232